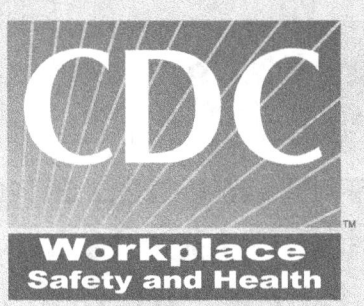

Ergonomic Evaluation at a Steel Grating Manufacturing Plant

Christine West, RN, MSN, MPH

Jessica Ramsey, MS

Health Hazard Evaluation Report
HETA 2008-0074-3081
Tru-Weld Grating, Inc.
Litchfield, Illinois
May 2009

DEPARTMENT OF HEALTH AND HUMAN SERVICES
Centers for Disease Control and Prevention

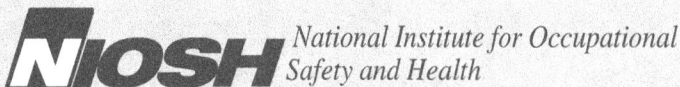

National Institute for Occupational Safety and Health

The employer shall post a copy of this report for a period of 30 calendar days at or near the workplace(s) of affected employees. The employer shall take steps to insure that the posted determinations are not altered, defaced, or covered by other material during such period. [37 FR 23640, November 7, 1972, as amended at 45 FR 2653, January 14, 1980].

CONTENTS

ABBREVIATIONS

BLS	Bureau of Labor Statistics
HHE	Health hazard evaluation
MSD	Musculoskeletal disorder
NAICS	North American Industry Classification System
NIOSH	National Institute for Occupational Safety and Health
OSHA	Occupational Safety and Health Administration
WMSD	Work-related musculoskeletal disorder

HIGHLIGHTS OF THE NIOSH HEALTH HAZARD EVALUATION

The National Institute for Occupational Safety and Health (NIOSH) received a joint union/ management request for a health hazard evaluation at Tru-Weld Grating Inc. in Litchfield, Illinois. The International Brotherhood of Boilermakers, Local 486 and Tru-Weld Grating Inc. management submitted the request due to high numbers of musculoskeletal disorders (MSDs) in employees working in the barline, welding, and saw areas. A site investigation was conducted in February 2008.

What NIOSH Did

- We observed and videotaped employees in the barline, welding, and saw areas to document risk factors for work-related musculoskeletal disorders (WMSDs). We also measured workstation heights and reach distances to determine injury risk.

- We asked employees about their work and medical history. We also asked about any history of WMSDs to determine the scope of the injuries that occur at the facility.

- We reviewed injury and illness logs and workers' compensation data.

- We compared rates of nonfatal injuries and illnesses in this workforce with national rates for ornamental and architectural metal work manufacturing facilities.

What NIOSH Found

- Employees are at an increased risk for WMSDs due to awkward postures, forceful exertions, and repetitive motions.

- Employees reported increased musculoskeletal pain and discomfort in their back and shoulders at work.

- Almost half of the injury and illness log entries recorded during the past 5 years were WMSDs. Most of these were in the shoulder and back.

- Rates of nonfatal injury and illness at Tru-Weld Grating are higher than in ornamental and architectural metal work manufacturing facilities nationally.

What Managers Can Do

- Design horizontal work surfaces (welding loading tables, saw area pallets, and catch basins) between heights of 28" and 56".

- Install powered roller conveyors in the saw areas and replace grooved surfaces at the saw tables with a smooth surface.

- Implement work practice changes, such as asking employees to grind welds instead of using a pry bar, walk around to adjust machine settings, and avoid leaning forward to clean scrap from the saw.

- Place antifatigue floor mats at each workstation to reduce worker fatigue from prolonged standing.

- Create a routine maintenance schedule for all equipment.

- Offer all employees ergonomics training.

- Encourage employees to report WMSDs to management and to seek care from a qualified provider.

- Encourage participation in the health and safety committee. Ask employees for ideas about how to prevent WMSDs.

- Decrease the amount of mandatory overtime for employees.

What Employees Can Do

- In the barline area, grind welds instead of prying them loose.

- Promptly report injuries or unsafe work conditions to management.

- Seek care from a healthcare provider knowledgeable about WMSDs.

- Take the time to work safely.

- Take part in ergonomic training.

- Take part in the health and safety committee and recommend ways to reduce WMSDs.

SUMMARY

NIOSH investigators conclude that a health hazard exists at the Tru-Weld Grating plant for employees working in the barline, welding, and saw areas. Employees in the barline, welding, and saw areas are exposed to a combination of risk factors for WMSDs in the upper extremities and back due to awkward postures, forceful exertions, and repetitive motions. Review of injury and illness records show lost workdays for MSDs and higher incidence rates of nonfatal injury and illness at Tru-Weld Grating than in the same type of facilities nationally. Recommendations for reducing the risk of WMSDs are included in this report, such as the use of adjustable tables and improved workplace design.

On December 14, 2007, NIOSH received a joint union/ management request for an HHE at Tru-Weld Grating Inc. in Litchfield, Illinois. The International Brotherhood of Boilermakers, Local 486 and management at Tru-Weld Grating submitted the request to investigate the high number of MSDs in employees working in the barline, welding, and saw areas.

On February 19–20, 2008, NIOSH investigators conducted an evaluation. The NIOSH ergonomist observed and videotaped job tasks in the work areas. The NIOSH epidemiologist conducted confidential health interviews with employees at the plant, reviewed OSHA's Form 300 Log of Work-Related Injuries and Illnesses (OSHA Logs), analyzed incidence rates from the OSHA Logs for the past 5 years, and reviewed employees' compensation data for the past 4 years.

NIOSH investigators observed that most employees are exposed to risk factors for developing WMSDs due to awkward postures, forceful exertions, and repetitive motions. These included prying materials loose with pry bars, squatting and bending over at the waist and back to maneuver heavy materials, reaching at or above shoulder height, and manipulating material using awkward shoulder and wrist postures.

The OSHA Logs and employees' compensation data review indicated that most WMSDs during the past 5 years (2003–2007) involved the back and shoulder, resulting in 698 days away from work and 49 days on job transfer or job restriction. The most common job involving WMSDs on the OSHA Logs and employees' compensation reports was Machine Operator (11), and the most common work location was on the #2 and #3 welders (7). We calculated the following injury/illness incidence rates from the OSHA Logs at the Tru-Weld Grating plant: 13.0 in 2003, 19.5 in 2004, 15.8 in 2005, 36.0 in 2006, and 24.3 in 2007 per 100 full-time employees. Incidence rates of nonfatal injury and illness were higher at the Tru-Weld Grating plant than incidence rates for ornamental and architectural metal work manufacturing facilities nationally from 2003–2007.

Of the 26 employees interviewed, 12 employees (60%) from the barline, welding, and saw areas reported 20 upper and lower extremity musculoskeletal symptoms that were worse at work. The most common areas where musculoskeletal symptoms were reported were the shoulder (5) and back (5). Employees also reported working mandatory overtime, missing work, seeing a healthcare provider, and transferring to different departments because of MSDs.

Keywords: NAICS 332323 (Ornamental and Architectural Metal Work Manufacturing), ergonomics, repetitive motions, work-related musculoskeletal disorders, pulling, reaching

INTRODUCTION

On December 14, 2007, NIOSH received a joint union/ management request for an HHE at Tru-Weld Grating Inc. in Litchfield, Illinois. The International Brotherhood of Boilermakers, Local 486, and management at Tru-Weld Grating submitted the request to investigate the high number of MSDs. Prior to the site visit, management and union representatives identified three areas (barline, welding, and saw) where they perceived most injuries were occurring.

On February 19–20, 2008, an ergonomist and epidemiologist from NIOSH conducted an evaluation at the Tru-Weld Grating plant. On February 19, 2008, NIOSH investigators held an opening conference with management and a representative from the International Brotherhood of Boilermakers, Local 486. NIOSH investigators toured the manufacturing areas and observed tasks occurring in the barline, welding, and saw areas of the plant. In addition, NIOSH investigators conducted confidential health interviews with employees, reviewed the OSHA Form 300 Log of Work-Related Injuries and Illnesses (OSHA Logs), analyzed nonfatal injury and illness incidence rates from the OSHA Logs, and reviewed employees' compensation data for the past 5 years. On February 20, 2008, NIOSH investigators held a closing conference and provided preliminary recommendations to the union and management representative.

Process Description

Tru-Weld Grating, owned by Fisher and Ludlow, manufactures steel grating for road bridges, industrial walkways, sidewalk vent covers, and other applications. The company receives spools of raw steel (3–4 feet wide), runs the steel through a slitter machine that cuts it down to various widths (1–3 inches), and respools it. These spools of steel are loaded into barline machines that straighten and flatten the raw material, then cut it to length. Steel rods are twisted and then used as cross supports for the grate. The materials (bars and rods) are fed through hydraulic welders that weld the pieces into the grate. The grating is then cut to a specified length in the saw area. Forklifts and overhead cranes are used to transport all the steel spools and gratings through the plant. A fabrication shop welds and assembles smaller grating and custom pieces. The Tru-Weld Grating plant employs 60 personnel, with 22 working in the barline, welding, and saw areas. They work three shifts, 8 hours per shift, 5 days per week. Management places a signup sheet in the break room daily as needed for departments that will be working overtime. Employees can sign up for overtime; however, mandatory overtime is required to fill empty slots to obtain the required number of employees.

Job Descriptions

Barline

Tishken and Gassner manufacture the two barline machines used at the plant. The Tishken machine runs smaller bar, and the Gassner machine runs thicker/heavier bar. Material handlers deliver spools of material and load them on the barline machine. Employees on the barline machines pry or grind welds loose on new spools of material. They also use the grinder to smooth the welds on the roll. Barline employees then pull the material over to the barline machine, hammer it flat, and weld it to the end of the piece from the previous roll. The machine pulls the material through and cuts it to a specified size. A dump table drops the cut material into a stack. Material handlers remove the stack and either store it or take it to the welding area.

Welding

The two welding machines are referred to as #2 and #3. The #2 machine runs the smaller bar, and the #3 machine runs the heavier bar. Material handlers deliver cut material to the welding machines and place the cut bar on the loading table. One employee on the welding machine removes the bar from a loading table and places it into a comb rack that feeds into the welding machine; this is called "pitching bar." The other employee on the welding machine inspects the bar as it feeds into the welding machine and makes adjustments as necessary. These two employees rotate positions every 2 hours (at each break). The grating is cut to specifications, and the machine transfers it to a finished stack. Material handlers remove the finished, stacked grating and either store the grating or take it to the saw areas.

Saw Areas

We observed two saw areas in the plant; each had one saw. Material handlers deliver grating to the saw areas and place it on sawhorses. Employees in the saw areas use a jib crane to load the grating on a roller conveyor. Saw employees push and pull grating toward the saw, then cut the grating to the specified size. The employees in the saw areas then use a jib crane to place the cut pieces on pallets on the floor. Material handlers remove the pallets of finished grating and either store the grating or take it to the fabrication area.

We walked through the Tru-Weld Grating plant to observe the processes of loading, machining, and fabricating to produce the steel grating product. Our observations focused on three areas of the plant identified by the management and union, the barline, welding, and saw areas where raw steel material is cut, welded, and prepared for fabrication. We took digital videos to document the tasks performed by the employees and measured workstation heights. We considered WMSDs as those MSDs to which the work environment and the performance of work contribute significantly, or MSDs that are made worse or longer lasting by work conditions. A full description of the ergonomics evaluation criteria we used to determine risk factors for WMSDs is provided in Appendix A.

We reviewed the number and types of injuries and illnesses from the OSHA Logs for years 2003–2007 and employees' compensation reports for 2004–2007. Nonfatal injury and illness and WMSD incidence rates were calculated from the OSHA Logs for years 2003–2007. Nonfatal injury and illness rates at the Tru-Weld Grating plant were compated to national incidence rates for ornamental and architectural metal work manufacturing facilities for years 2003–2007 (NAICS code: 332323). This calculation and comparison were performed using a formula available on the BLS website at http://data bls.gov/IIRC/calculate.do. WMSD national incidence rates were not available for comparison.

The incidence rate of injuries and illnesses is determined by multiplying the number of injuries and illnesses (or number of WMSDs) by 200,000 and dividing this number by the number of actual employee hours worked per year. The 200,000 hours in the formula represents the equivalent of 100 employees working 40 hours per week, 50 weeks per year and provides the standard base for the incidence rates.

The NIOSH epidemiologist interviewed 26 employees in a private setting; all employees from the barline, #2 and #3 welders, and saw areas were selected for interviews. Eight additional employees were serially selected from an employee roster for the other areas of the plant (serrator, slitter, maintenance, grating fabrication, and general production). Interview questions concerned personal characteristics, medical history, job duties, and MSDs. Employees were asked if they had pain, aching, stiffness, burning, numbness, and other symptoms indicative of MSDs during the past year. Employees were also asked to identify the location, characteristics, and severity of the symptom(s).

Barline

One employee runs each barline machine; we observed employees at both barline machines. We noted that employees were prying welds loose using a pry bar instead of using the grinder as preferred by Tru-Weld Grating plant management. The degree of force required to remove the weld depends on the size of the weld. Employees in the slitter area are asked to make as small a weld as possible to eliminate excessive force to remove welds. NIOSH investigators observed barline employees leaning over machines to make adjustments that keep the bar on the dump table. Management has asked them to walk around the machine to make these adjustments to eliminate extended reaches and awkward back postures. Also, for material handlers removing finished material, the bottom of the catch basin was measured at 15″, requiring material handlers to squat and bend over at the waist to place chains around the material before using the overhead crane to move it.

Welding

We observed employees at both welding machines. We noted that employees on the #2 welder had to reach at or above shoulder height to retrieve the bar from the loading table. Height measurements taken at the #2 welder were 31″ at the comb rack and 46″–56″ at the loading table. We also noted that employees on the #3 welder had to bend at the back to place the bar into the comb rack. Height measurements taken at the #3 welder were 27″ at the comb rack and 41″–48″ at the loading table. Additionally, some of the thinner material became tangled on the loading table and employees flipped it to untangle, causing awkward shoulder and wrist postures.

Saw Areas

One employee runs each saw; we observed employees at both saw areas. We noted that employees used jib cranes to lift grating from pallets and lower the grating to the roller conveyor. The health and safety specialist for the union recently suggested replacing the roller conveyor in the saw area. This had been completed prior to our site visit, and employees commented that it made moving the grating on the conveyor somewhat easier. However, because of the size and weight of the grating, employees still use pry bars to push and pull the grating down the conveyor. We also noted that the material gets hung up when it gets closer to the saw because the roller conveyor ends, and the saw table has grooves (probably from wear). The employees also sweep away the scrap material when cleaning the end of the grating piece. A catch basin was observed under each saw table; however, the employees leaned over and swept the scrap into their hands and then carried it to the dumpster. The cut grating is stored on pallets directly on the floor, requiring the employee to bend at the waist and squat to maneuver the grating into the proper position.

OSHA Logs

Of 56 recordable injuries recorded on the OSHA Logs between 2003 and 2007 (excluding fractures, contusions, or lacerations), 24 were WMSDs (43%). The most common WMSD recorded was back pain/strain (10) and shoulder strain/pull (9). The other WMSDs recorded were elbow pain/strain (2), wrist pain/strain (2), and foot strain (1). The most common occupation of employees who reported WMSDs was Machine Operator, and the most common location where the WMSD occurred was on the #2 and #3 welders. The number of WMSDs varied from three to five (43% to 63%) in 2003–2005. In 2006, eight WSMDs were recorded (40%); five (33%) were recorded in 2007. A total of 698 days away from work and 49 days on job transfer or job restriction were reported for WMSD injuries from 2003–2007.

Table 1 compares incidence rates of nonfatal injuries and illnesses at the Tru-Weld Grating plant to incidence rates for ornamental and architectural metal work manufacturing facilities nationally from 2003–2007. Nonfatal injury and illness incidence rates at the plant were higher than national rates from 2003–2007. WMSD incidence rates were variable from 2003–2007. WMSD national incidence rates were not available for comparison.

Table 1. Comparison of Nonfatal Injury and Illness Incidence Rates at Tru-Weld Grating to Ornamental and Architectural Metal Work Manufacturing Facilities Nationally, 2003–2007

Year	Incidence Rates* at Tru-Weld Grating	WMSD Incidence Rates[†] at Tru-Weld Grating	National Incidence Rates[‡]
2003	13.0	6.5	11.1
2004	19.5	12.2	7.4
2005	15.8	6.8	10.3
2006	36.0	14.4	8.5
2007	24.3	8.1	10.3

*Incidence rate = (number of injuries and illnesses × 200,000)/employee hours worked
[†] WMSD incidence rate = (number of WMSDs × 200,000)/employee hours worked
[‡] U.S. ornamental and architectural metal work manufacturing facilities (NAICS code: 332323)

Employees' Compensation Data

Employees filed five employees' compensation claims for WMSDs in 2004, six in 2005, nine in 2006, and four in 2007. The WMSDs with the largest number of claims were shoulder strain (8) and back strain (8). The most common occupation given was Machine Operator (11), and most common work location was on the #2 and #3 welders (7).

Health Interviews

We interviewed 26 employees. The average job duration reported was 12 years (range: 1 month–31 years), and the average age was 40 years (range: 19–55). The interviews included 18 employees from the barline, welding, and saw areas and 8 employees from other areas of the plant. Twelve employees (60%) from the barline, welding, and saw areas reported musculoskeletal symptoms at multiple sites. Of the musculoskeletal symptoms reported, the most common were in the shoulder (5) and back (5). Of those interviewed from the other plant areas, four employees reported upper and lower extremity musculoskeletal symptoms. Three employees reported being diagnosed with carpal tunnel syndrome, two reported a diagnosis of tendonitis, and one reported a diagnosis of cubital tunnel syndrome. Other reported evidence of musculoskeletal symptoms included eight employees seeing a healthcare provider, seven employees missing work, and two employees transferring to a different department because of musculoskeletal symptoms. Most of the employees reported they are required to work overtime, which typically includes an 8-hour shift on the weekend.

Health and Safety Committee Meetings

Management and employees reported that a health and safety committee at Tru-Weld Grating holds monthly meetings to discuss safety issues. Employees reported that they thought meetings were not held frequently enough, safety issues were not resolved quickly, and that health and safety issues could not be raised until the meetings were held.

DISCUSSION

We found that employees in the barline, welding, and saw areas are exposed to a combination of concurrent risk factors for developing upper WMSDs, including awkward postures, forceful exertions, and repetitive motions. Likewise, employees also had exposure to factors associated with back injuries, including lifting, squatting, twisting movements of the trunk, and bending at the waist. We also observed and documented that employees were at risk for WMSDs in the shoulder and back. Working at or above shoulder level, flipping material, prying, and pushing have strong associations with shoulder WMSDs. These combinations of work factors leading to neck/shoulder MSDs and back pain/strain have been documented in previous studies [Holmström et al. 1992; NIOSH 1997; Miranda et al. 2001]. A number of personal factors such as age, sex, smoking, physical activity, and strength can also influence the occurrence of MSDs [NIOSH 1997].

The interviews, OSHA Logs, and employees' compensation data confirmed that the most common WMSD injuries reported were to the shoulder and back. The most common occupation listed on the OSHA Logs and employees' compensation reports was Machine Operator, and the most common work location for MSDs to occur was in the area of the #2 and #3 welders. Of those interviewed who worked in the barline, welding, and saw areas, a higher percentage of employees reported WMSDs than in the other areas. In addition, most of the employees reported working overtime. Several studies have found an association between working overtime (working more than 8 hours per day or more than 40 hours per week) and development of WMSDs. Overtime not only lengthens the time an employee is exposed to known risk factors, but can contribute to fatigue, impaired performance, and stress that can lead to a risk of unintentional injuries [Bergqvist et al. 1995; Fredriksson et al. 1999; Dembe et al. 2005].

Higher incidence rates of all nonfatal injury and illness were found at Tru-Weld Grating when compared to national rates of nonfatal injury and illness for ornamental and architectural metal work manufacturing facilities from 2003–2007. We also calculated WMSD incidence rates to better understand the impact of the WMSDs in this particular workplace. The rates of nonfatal injury and illnesses and WMSDs varied during the 5-year time period. The incidence rates from the OSHA Logs provide an estimate of the magnitude of injuries and illnesses occurring at the plant and of WMSDs occurring at the plant. We believe that WMSDs may have been underreported in the OSHA Logs as evidenced

DISCUSSION
(CONTINUED)

by more than half of the employees interviewed reporting MSD symptoms and the number of employees' compensation claims for WMSDs exceeding the number of WMSDs reported in the OSHA Logs in 2006 and 2007. This is consistent with other evidence of underreporting WMSDs in the U.S. workforce [Morse et al. 2005]. Although incidence rates at Tru-Weld Grating were higher than national incidence rates, the rates at Tru-Weld Grating may be unstable due to the small size of this workforce. Rates based on small numbers may fluctuate from year to year or differ considerably, even when there might be no meaningful difference.

CONCLUSIONS

Employees in the barline, welding, and saw areas are exposed to a combination of risk factors for WMSDs in the upper extremities due to awkward postures, forceful exertions, and repetitive motions and in the back due to lifting, squatting, twisting movements of the trunk, and bending at the waist. Employees reported shoulder and back pain, working mandatory overtime, missing work, seeing a healthcare provider, and transferring to different departments because of WMSDs. We believe that the combination of these factors is contributing to an increased risk of WMSDs at Tru-Weld Grating compared to the same type of facilities (ornamental and architectural metal work manufacturing) nationally.
Review of the OSHA Logs shows lost workdays from WMSDs. Recommendations for reducing the risk of WMSDs such as the use of adjustable tables and improved workplace design, are included in this report.

RECOMMENDATIONS

The following recommendations are offered to help reduce the risk of WMSDs for employees at Tru-Weld Grating. The preferred method of controlling workplace risk factors for WMSDs is to provide engineering controls that redesign the workstation and/or job task. Administrative controls are designed to limit employees' exposures to hazardous conditions and can be used temporarily until engineering controls are implemented. The effectiveness of administrative changes in work practices for controlling WMSDs depends on management commitment and employee acceptance. In addition, recommendations are given to change work practices, improve healthcare management, and to encourage active employee participation in the health and safety committee to reduce WMSDs.

Engineering Controls

General recommendations for engineering controls that would eliminate or significantly reduce physical stresses in individual areas are listed below.

- Design all work areas within a working height range of 28" to 56" [Kroemer 1989]. The current measurements of the welding area are near the top of this range. Moving the working height toward the middle of the range should reduce the risk for back and shoulder WMSDs. This same height range should be incorporated for the finished material in the barline and saw areas to eliminate bending at the back and squatting.

- Install a powered roller conveyor in the saw area to eliminate pushing and pulling forces required to move grating on the conveyor.

- Install additional rollers next to the saw tables and replace the saw tables' grooved surfaces with smooth surfaces. This should improve push/pull forces and eliminate material getting caught and requiring excessive push forces.

Administrative Controls

Administrative control recommendations for all processes/areas include those listed below. Regular monitoring and reinforcement are necessary to ensure that control policies and procedures are not circumvented in the name of convenience, schedule, or production. Employee training should complement efforts to address workplace safety and health problems, including those focused on workplace risk factors for WMSDs and related concerns [NIOSH 1997].

- Rotate employees through several jobs with different physical demands to reduce the stress on limbs and body regions.

- Schedule more breaks to allow for rest and recovery. Taking short breaks for 3–5 minutes every hour can give the body a rest and reduce discomfort.

- Minimize the use of mandatory overtime by hiring more employees, rotating employees off shifts, and allowing weekend recovery time more consistently.

- Broaden or vary job content to offset certain WMSD risk factors including repetitive motions, forceful exertions, static and awkward postures.

- Provide additional training in ergonomics for supervisors and members of the health and safety committee. If the plant cannot provide this training for all health and safety committee members, the head of the health and safety committee should receive additional ergonomics training because he/she has overall responsibility for this committee.

- Train employees to recognize WMSDs and instruct them in work practices that can ease the task demands or burden.

- Continue performing job hazard analyses but include the evaluation of WMSD risk factors. Encourage active involvement of employees in these evaluations. Perform job analyses on any new process or when new equipment is introduced.

- Implement the use of an ergonomic checklist and referral form. Checklists can offer an orderly procedure for screening jobs for risk factors of consequence to WMSDs. Examples of checklists from NIOSH document, *Elements of Ergonomics Programs: A Primer Based on Evaluations of Musculoskeletal Disorders* are given in Appendix B; these lists can be customized to fit the needs and issues of the workforce at Tru-Weld Grating [NIOSH 1997b]. Additional checklists can be found on the NIOSH website at www.cdc.gov/niosh/docs/97-117/epchklst.html.

Work Practices

Changing how employees perform specific tasks can also significantly reduce risks of WMSDs. Developing standard operating procedures can help achieve this goal.

- Ensure that employees in the barline area are grinding welds, not prying them loose. To facilitate this, ensure that employees in the slitter area are aware of using a minimal weld that can be easily removed by barline employees.

- Ensure that employees in the barline area are walking around the machines to make adjustments. This eliminates extended reaches and the risk of low back and shoulder injuries.

Recommendations
(CONTINUED)

- Remind employees in the saw area to use a small hand broom to sweep scrap into the catch basin rather than leaning and sweeping it into their hands. This will also eliminate extended reaches and lower the risk of back and shoulder WMSDs.

- Equip all areas with antifatigue floor mats and/or foot rests to reduce muscle fatigue and low back pain from prolonged standing. Special material may be required to reduce the potential for slip and fall injuries where oils are present.

- Keep equipment, such as jib cranes and conveyor systems, well maintained and in proper working order. Implement an active routine maintenance system.

Healthcare Management

Healthcare management emphasizes the prevention of impairment and disability through early detection, prompt treatment, and timely recovery. Healthcare management recommendations include the following:

- Encourage employees to report musculoskeletal symptoms to their supervisors and management and to seek a prompt referral to a healthcare provider experienced in the evaluation and treatment of WMSDs. If symptoms are identified and treated early, it is less likely that a more serious disorder will develop.

- Consistently record cases of WMSDs on OSHA Logs and other incident reporting systems to analyze trends and understand the magnitude and seriousness of WMSDs. These records may also offer leads to jobs or operations that can cause or contribute to WMSDs.

- Provide education and training to employees regarding recognition of the symptoms and signs of WMSDs and the employer's procedures for reporting WMSDs.

Health and Safety Committee

Management and employees working together to identify work hazards and propose ergonomic solutions is a key component to a successful health and safety committee. The following

RECOMMENDATIONS
(CONTINUED)

recommendations should improve the responsiveness of the existing health and safety committee at Tru-Weld Grating to the ergonomic needs of employees.

- Encourage the existing health and safety committee consisting of management and employee representatives to develop a written health and safety program that is endorsed by management and employee representatives and communicated to all employees. The program should consist of procedures and mechanisms to identify and evaluate ergonomic health and safety hazards.

- Health and safety committee meetings should be held regularly to evaluate progress, assign responsibilities, and identify potential problem areas. Along with covering health and safety topics at the meetings, ergonomic issues should also be discussed. However, if employees have immediate health and safety concerns, they should be raised and addressed at any time between the meetings.

REFERENCES

Bergqvist U, Wolgast E, Nilsson B, Voss M [1995]. Musculoskeletal disorders among visual display terminal employees: individual, ergonomic, and work organizational factors. Ergonomics 38(4):763–776.

Dembe AE, Erickson JB, Delbos RG, Banks SM [2005]. The impact of overtime and long work hours on occupational injuries and illnesses: new evidence from the United States. Occup Environ Med 62(9):588–597.

Fredriksson K, Alfredsson L, Köster M, Thorbjörnsson CB, Toomingas A, Torgén M, Kilbom A [1999]. Risk factors for neck and upper limb disorders: results from 24 years of follow up. Occup Environ Med 56(1):59–66.

Holmström EB, Lindell J, Moritz U [1992]. Low back and neck/shoulder pain in construction employees: occupational workload and psychosocial risk factors. Part 2: Relationship to neck and shoulder pain. Spine 17(6):672–677.

Kroemer KHE [1989]. Engineering anthropometry. Ergonomics 32(7):767–784.

REFERENCES
(CONTINUED)

Miranda H, Viikari-Juntura E, Martikainen R, Takala EP, Riihimäki H [2001]. A prospective study of work related factors and physical exercise as predictors of shoulder pain. Occup Environ Med 58(8):528–534.

Morse T, Dillon C, Kenta-Bibi E, Weber J, Diva U, Warren N, Grey M [2005]. Trends in work-related musculoskeletal disorder reports by year, type, and industrial sector: a capture-recapture analysis. Am J Ind Med 48(1):40–49.

NIOSH [1997]. Musculoskeletal disorders and workplace factors: a critical review of epidemiologic evidence for work-related musculoskeletal disorders of the neck, upper extremity, and low back. Cincinnati, OH: U.S. Department of Health and Human Services, Centers for Disease Control and Prevention, National Institute for Occupational Safety and Health, (DHHS) Publication No. 97-141. [www.cdc.gov/niosh/docs/97-141/].

Musculoskeletal disorders are those conditions that involve the nerves, tendons, muscles, and supporting structures of the body. They can be characterized by chronic pain and limited mobility. WMSD refers to (1) musculoskeletal disorders to which the work environment and the performance of work contribute significantly, or (2) MSDs that are made worse or longer lasting by work conditions. A substantial body of data provides strong evidence of an association between MSDs and certain work-related factors (physical, work organizational, psychosocial, individual, and sociocultural). The multifactorial nature of MSDs requires a discussion of individual factors and how they are associated with WMSDs. Strong evidence shows that working groups with high levels of static contraction, prolonged static loads, or extreme working postures involving the neck/shoulder muscles are at increased risk for neck/shoulder MSDs [NIOSH 1997a]. Further strong evidence shows job tasks that require a combination of risk factors (highly repetitious, forceful hand/wrist exertions) increase risk for hand/wrist tendonitis [NIOSH 1997a]. Lastly, strong evidence shows that low-back disorders are associated with work-related lifting and forceful movements [NIOSH 1997a]. A number of personal factors can also influence the response to risk factors for MSDs: age, sex, smoking, physical activity, strength, and anthropometry. Although personal factors may affect an individual's susceptibility to overexertion injuries/disorders, studies conducted in high-risk industries show that the risk associated with personal factors is small compared to that associated with occupational exposures [NIOSH 1997a].

In all cases, the preferred method for preventing and controlling WMSDs is to design jobs, workstations, tools, and other equipment to match the physiological, anatomical, and psychological characteristics and capabilities of the employee. Under these conditions, exposures to risk factors considered potentially hazardous are reduced or eliminated.

The specific criteria used to evaluate jobs at Tru-Weld Grating were workplace and job design criteria found in the NIOSH document, *Elements of Ergonomic Programs: A Primer Based on Evaluations of Musculoskeletal Disorders* [NIOSH 1997b].

Workstation design should directly relate to the anatomical characteristics of the employee. Because a variety of employees may use a specific workstation, a range of work heights should be considered. Based upon female/male 50th and 95th percentile anthropometric data, workstation heights should be within a range of 28" to no higher than 60" [Kroemer 1989]. These heights correspond to knuckle and shoulder dimensions of United States civilians, age 20 to 60 years.

References

Kroemer KHE [1989]. Engineering anthropometry. Ergonomics 32(7):767–784.

NIOSH [1997a]. Musculoskeletal disorders and workplace factors: a critical review of epidemiologic evidence for work-related musculoskeletal disorders of the neck, upper extremity, and low back. Cincinnati, OH: U.S. Department of Health and Human Services, Centers for Disease Control and Prevention, National Institute for Occupational Safety and Health, (DHHS) Publication No. 97–141. [www.cdc.gov/niosh/docs/97-141/].

NIOSH [1997b]. Elements of ergonomic programs: a primer based on evaluations of musculoskeletal disorders. Cincinnati, OH: U.S. Department of Health and Human Services, Centers for Disease Control and Prevention, National Institute for Occupational Safety and Health, (DHHS) Publication No. 97–117. [www.cdc.gov/niosh/97-117pd.html].

1. General Ergonomic Risk Analysis Checklist*

Shade the dot if your answer is "yes" to the question. A "yes" response indicates that an ergonomic risk factor may be present which requires further analysis.

Manual Material Handling

- Is there lifting of loads, tools, or parts?
- Is there lowering of tools, loads, or parts?
- Is there overhead reaching for tools, loads, or parts?
- Is there bending at the waist to handle tools, loads, or parts?
- Is there twisting at the waist to handle tools, loads, or parts?

For further analysis, refer to checklist 5–F.

Physical Energy Demands

- Do tools and parts weigh more than 10 lb?
- Is reaching greater than 20 in.?
- Is bending, stooping, or squatting a primary task activity?
- Is lifting or lowering loads a primary task activity?
- Is walking or carrying loads a primary task activity?
- Is stair or ladder climbing with loads a primary task activity?
- Is pushing or pulling loads a primary task activity?
- Is reaching overhead a primary task activity?
- Do any of the above tasks require five or more complete work cycles to be done within a minute?
- Do employees complain that rest breaks and fatigue allowances are insufficient?

For further analysis, refer to checklist 5–F.

Other Musculoskeletal Demands

- Do manual jobs require frequent, repetitive motions?
- Do work postures require frequent bending of the neck, shoulder, elbow, wrist, or finger joints?
- For seated work, do reaches for tools and materials exceed 15 in. from the employee's position?
- Is the employee unable to change his or her position often?
- Does the work involve forceful, quick, or sudden motions?
- Does the work involve shock or rapid buildup of forces?
- Is finger-pinch gripping used?
- Do job postures involve sustained muscle contraction of any limb?

For further analysis, refer to checklists 5–C, 5–D, and 5–E.

Computer Workstation

- Do operators use computer workstations for more than 4 hours a day?
- Are there complaints of discomfort from those working at these stations?
- Is the chair or desk nonadjustable?
- Is the display monitor, keyboard, or document holder nonadjustable?
- Does lighting cause glare or make the monitor screen hard to read?
- Is the room temperature too hot or too cold?
- Is there irritating vibration or noise?

For further analysis, refer to checklist 5–G.

Environment

- Is the temperature too hot or too cold?
- Are the employee's hands exposed to temperatures less than 70 degrees Fahrenheit?
- Is the workplace poorly lit?
- Is there glare?
- Is there excessive noise that is annoying, distracting, or producing hearing loss?
- Is there upper extremity or whole body vibration?
- Is air circulation too high or too low?

General Workplace

- Are walkways uneven, slippery, or obstructed?
- Is housekeeping poor?
- Is there inadequate clearance or accessibility for performing tasks?
- Are stairs cluttered or lacking railings?
- Is proper footwear worn?

Tools

- Is the handle too small or too large?
- Does the handle shape cause the operator to bend the wrist in order to use the tool?
- Is the tool hard to access?
- Does the tool weigh more than 9 lb?
- Does the tool vibrate excessively?
- Does the tool cause excessive kickback to the operator?
- Does the tool become too hot or too cold?

For further analysis, refer to checklist 5–E.

Gloves

- Do the gloves require the employee to use more force when performing job tasks?
- Do the gloves provide inadequate protection?
- Do the gloves present a hazard of catch points on the tool or in the workplace?

Administration

- Is there little employee control over the work process?
- Is the task highly repetitive and monotonous?
- Does the job involve critical tasks with high accountability and little or no tolerance for error?
- Are work hours and breaks poorly organized?

*Adapted from The University of Utah Research Foundation "Checklist for General Ergonomic Risk Analysis," available from the ERGOWEB Internet site (http://ergoweb.com/).

2. Ergonomic Hazard Identification Checklist

Answer the following questions based on the primary job activities of employees in this facility.

Use the following responses to describe how frequently employees are exposed to the job conditions described below:

Never (employee is never exposed to the condition)
Sometimes (employee is exposed to the condition less than 3 times daily)
Usually (employee is exposed to the condition 3 times or more daily)

	Never	Sometimes	Usually	If USUALLY, list jobs to which answer applies here
1. Do employees perform tasks that are externally paced?				
2. Are employees required to exert force with their hands (e.g., gripping, pulling, pinching)?				
3. Do employees use handtools or handle parts or objects?				
4. Do employees stand continuously for periods of more than 30 min?				
5. Do employees sit for periods of more than 30 min without the opportunity to stand or move around freely?				
6. Do employees use electronic input devices (e.g., keyboards, mice, joysticks, track balls) for continuous periods of more than 30 min?				
7. Do employees kneel (one or both knees)?				
8. Do employees perform activities with hands raised above shoulder height?				
9. Do employees perform activities while bending or twisting at the waist?				
10. Are employees exposed to vibration?				
11. Do employees lift or lower objects between floor and waist height or above shoulder height?				
12. Do employees lift or lower objects more than once per min for continuous periods of more than 15 min?				
13. Do employees lift, lower, or carry large objects or objects that cannot be held close to the body?				
14. Do employees lift, lower, or carry objects weighing more than 50 lb?				

GLOSSARY OF TERMS

Facility: The location to which employees report each day for work. For situations in which employees do not report to any fixed location on a regular basis but are subject to common supervision, the facility may be defined as a central location where other OSHA records are maintained. (Note: Synonymous with establishment, as defined in OSHA record keeping requirements.)

Primary job activities: Job activities that make up a significant part of the work or are required for safety or contingency. Activities are not considered to be primary job activities if they makeup a small percentage of the job (i.e., take up less than 10% of the employee's time), are not essential for safety or contingency, and can be readily accomplished in other ways (e.g., using equipment already available in the facility).

Externally paced activities: Work activities for which the employee does not have direct control of the rate of work. Externally paced work activities include activities for which (1) the employee must keep up with an assembly line or an independently-operating machine, (2) the employee must respond to a continuous queue (e.g., customers standing in line, phone calls at a switchboard), or (3) time standards are imposed on employees.

3. Task Analysis Checklist

"No" responses indicate potential problem areas which should receive further investigation.		
1. Does the design of the primary task reduce or eliminate		
bending or twisting of the back or trunk?	[ ]yes	[ ]no
crouching?	[ ]yes	[ ]no
bending or twisting the wrist?	[ ]yes	[ ]no
extending the arms?	[ ]yes	[ ]no
raised elbows?	[ ]yes	[ ]no
static muscle loading?	[ ]yes	[ ]no
clothes wringing motions?	[ ]yes	[ ]no
finger pinch grip?	[ ]yes	[ ]no
2. Are mechanical devices used when necessary?	[ ]yes	[ ]no
3. Can the task be done with either hand?	[ ]yes	[ ]no
4. Can the task be done with two hands?	[ ]yes	[ ]no
5. Are pushing or pulling forces kept minimal?	[ ]yes	[ ]no
6. Are required forces judged acceptable by the employees?	[ ]yes	[ ]no
7. Are the materials		
able to be held without slipping?	[ ]yes	[ ]no
easy to grasp?	[ ]yes	[ ]no
free from sharp edges and corners?	[ ]yes	[ ]no
8. Do containers have good handholds?	[ ]yes	[ ]no
9. Are jigs, fixtures, and vises used where needed?	[ ]yes	[ ]no
10. As needed, do gloves fit properly and are they made of the proper fabric?	[ ]yes	[ ]no
11. Does the employee avoid contact with sharp edges when performing the task?	[ ]yes	[ ]no
12. When needed, are push buttons designed properly?	[ ]yes	[ ]no
13. Do the job tasks allow for ready use of personal equipment that may be required?	[ ]yes	[ ]no
14. Are high rates of repetitive motion avoided by		
job rotation?	[ ]yes	[ ]no
self-pacing?	[ ]yes	[ ]no
sufficient pauses?	[ ]yes	[ ]no
adjusting the job skill level of the employee?	[ ]yes	[ ]no
15. Is the employee trained in		
proper work practices?	[ ]yes	[ ]no
when and how to make adjustments?	[ ]yes	[ ]no
recognizing signs and symptoms of potential problems?	[ ]yes	[ ]no

ACKNOWLEDGMENTS AND AVAILABILITY OF REPORT

The Hazard Evaluations and Technical Assistance Branch (HETAB) of the National Institute for Occupational Safety and Health (NIOSH) conducts field investigations of possible health hazards in the workplace. These investigations are conducted under the authority of Section 20(a)(6) of the Occupational Safety and Health (OSHA) Act of 1970, 29 U.S.C. 669(a)(6) which authorizes the Secretary of Health and Human Services, following a written request from any employer or authorized representative of employees, to determine whether any substance normally found in the place of employment has potentially toxic effects in such concentrations as used or found. HETAB also provides, upon request, technical and consultative assistance to federal, state, and local agencies; labor; industry; and other groups or individuals to control occupational health hazards and to prevent related trauma and disease.

The findings and conclusions in this report are those of the authors and do not necessarily represent the views of NIOSH. Mention of any company or product does not constitute endorsement by NIOSH. In addition, citations to websites external to NIOSH do not constitute NIOSH endorsement of the sponsoring organizations or their programs or products. Furthermore, NIOSH is not responsible for the content of these websites. All Web addresses referenced in this document were accessible as of the publication date.

This report was prepared by Christine West and Jessica Ramsey of HETAB, Division of Surveillance, Hazard Evaluations and Field Studies. Health communication assistance was provided by Stefanie Evans. Editorial assistance was provided by Ellen Galloway. Desktop publishing was performed by Robin Smith.

Copies of this report have been sent to the president of the International Brotherhood of Boilermakers, Local 486, management representatives at Tru-Weld Grating, Inc., and the OSHA Regional Office. This report is not copyrighted and may be freely reproduced. The report may be viewed and printed at www.cdc.gov/niosh/hhe. Copies may be purchased from the National Technical Information Service at 5825 Port Royal Road, Springfield, Virginia 22161.

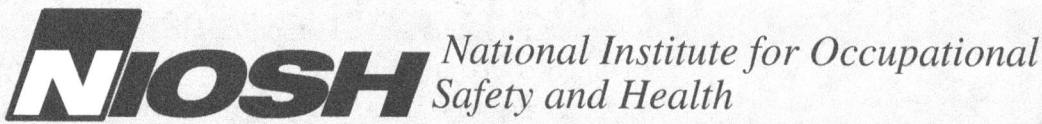

National Institute for Occupational
Safety and Health

Delivering on the Nation's promise:
Safety and health at work for all people
through research and prevention.

To receive NIOSH documents or information about
occupational safety and health topics, contact NIOSH at:

1-800-CDC-INFO (1-800-232-4636)

TTY: 1-888-232-6348

E-mail: cdcinfo@cdc.gov

or visit the NIOSH web site at: **www.cdc.gov/niosh.**

For a monthly update on news at NIOSH, subscribe to
NIOSH eNews by visiting **www.cdc.gov/niosh/eNews.**

SAFER • HEALTHIER • PEOPLE™